AIR FRYER COOKBOOK

Truly Healthy Fried Recipes with Low Salt and Low Fat, Ideal Cooking to Prevent Disease, Control Weight and Live Well While Eating. Keeps You and Your Family Healthy, Satisfies Splurges Without Any Guilt.

Violet H.Scott

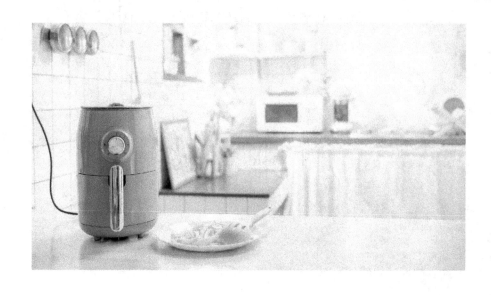

contained within this document, including, but not limited to, — errors, omissions, or inaccuracies.

Table of Contents

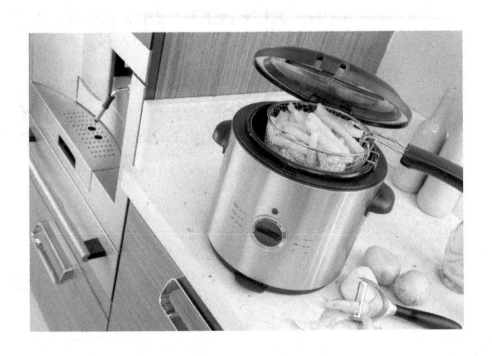

Introduction

Tired of depriving yourself of tasty fried foods because the pounds are adding up and your liver is screaming for help? The solution exists, and it is to use an air fryer- This is a fantastic and innovative appliance that makes it easy and fast to cook delicious and healthy meals,

that makes it easy and quick to cook delicious and healthy meals.

Easy to clean and store, convenience is one of its strengths.

Goodbye oil splatters, on the walls, on the floor. Not to mention the time it takes to deglaze the used product after cooking.

In a short period of time, the air fryer

will prepare your meal, whether it's chicken, steak, fish or vegetables,

frying them perfectly.

In addition to savory dishes, you can also use an air fryer with excellent results for cakes, tarts and even bread.

Its great advantage is the fact that it keeps the nutritional content intact compared to cooking with a classic fryer. High cooking temperatures deprive food of much of what our bodies need.

The difference is that when food is prepared in an air fryer, it is only cooked to the safe temperatures appropriate for your health and food. It prepares healthy meals with less time, more control and healthier results. It is the most efficient way to cook.

Hot air replaces oil, creating a crisp, delicious crust.

It will cook evenly, thanks to the perfect heat distribution aided by the fan.

The calories of typical fried foods will be a distant memory, with the absence or minimal amount of added oil, they will be reduced dramatically, without going to the expense of crispiness.

Your food will taste just like fried food, without the oil.

Equipped with a thermostat that comes with protection against overheating, there will be no danger of burning your food. There's also a food weight indicator, so you'll know the exact amount you're preparing, and a timer with an automatic shut-off feature, so you can safely do other activities while cooking.

Cooking takes place evenly, thanks to the perfect distribution of heat aided by the fan.

The calories of typical fried foods will be a distant memory, with the absence or minimal amount of oil added, will be reduced dramatically, without going to the expense of crispness.

Your food will taste just like fried food, without the oil.

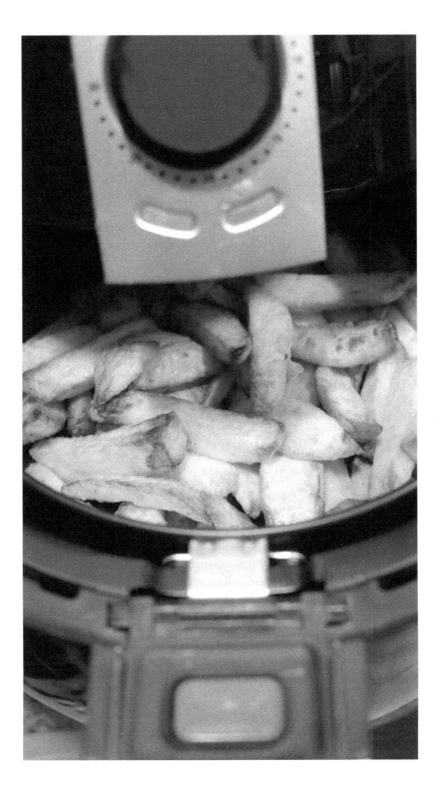

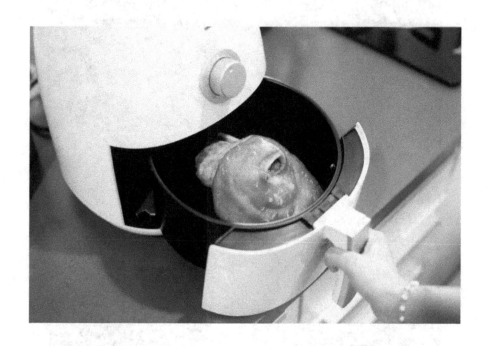

Air fryer recipes

PAPRIKA POTATO FRIES

To prepare

5 minutes

Prepare

20 minutes

Number of persons 4

Ingredients

750 gr sweet potato, about 4 pieces

1 tbsp chili powder

1 tbsp paprika powder

1 tbsp fine salt

Instructions

1. Heat the Airfryer to 180 ° C.

2. Peel the sweet potatoes and cut into equal slices of about 1 cm. Cut 1 cm wide fries from these slices.

3. Mix with chili powder, paprika and salt and bake in the Airfryer for 15 to 20 minutes.

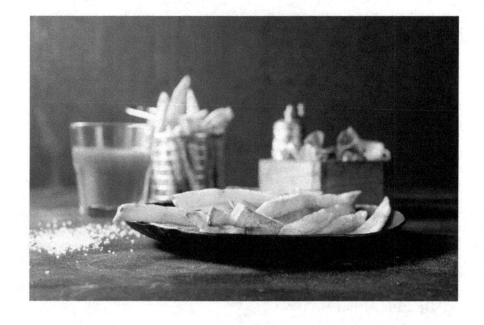

OVEN ZUCCHINI WITH SMOKED SALMON

Preparation time 15 minutes

Preparation time 45 minutes

Total time 1 hour

Ingredients

1 zucchini, at least 300 grams

200 grams of smoked salmon

3 tablespoons of mild olive oil

1 teaspoon of black pepper from the pepper mill

1/2 teaspoon of Celtic sea salt

1 large clove of garlic, finely chopped

80 grams créme fraiche

3 eggs, size large

75 grams of grated grana padano

☐handful of finely chopped fresh coriander

Instructions

Set your oven to 180 degrees to preheat. If you use an Airfryer, it also goes at 180 degrees.

Cut the zucchini into small cubes and the smoked salmon into strips.

In a frying pan, fry the garlic lightly brown in the mild olive oil and then add the zucchini cubes. Stir fry until the zucchini is almost cooked.

Turn off the heat and add the smoked salmon and coriander to the zucchini.

Meanwhile, in a bowl, stir together the eggs, creme fraiche and 50 grams of grana padano to a smooth batter.

Crumble your baking paper and place it in your baking tin.

Spoon the zucchini and smoked salmon mix into the baking tin. Pour the batter over it. Sprinkle the remaining 25 grams of Grana Padano over the quiche.

Bake in the center of the oven for 20-25 minutes.

If you use an Airfryer, the baking time is around 15 minutes at 180 degrees

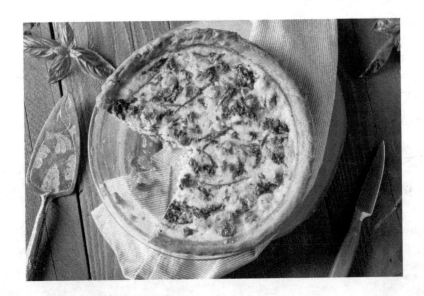

AIR FRYER HALLOUMI

Prep time 3 mins

Cook time 10 mins

Ingredients

1 lb halloumi (450 g)

½ cup breadcrumbs (8 tablespoons)

1 egg

½ teaspoon salt

½ teaspoon garlic powder

Instructions

Slice the halloumi into thick fries.

Crack the egg into a bowl, and whisk until it's combined. In another bowl, add the breadcrumbs, salt and garlic powder.

Use a fork to dip each halloumi stick individually into the whisked egg, then into the breadcrumbs. The cheese should be coated with the breading on all sides. Repeat with each fry.

Preheat your air fryer to 180 °C/ 355 °F. Then, add the breaded halloumi sticks to the air fryer basket. Make sure to leave room between each stick to allow the halloumi to cook evenly.

Air fry the halloumi fries for 8-10 minutes, turning them once halfway through the cooking time. Serve them immediately while they are still hot.

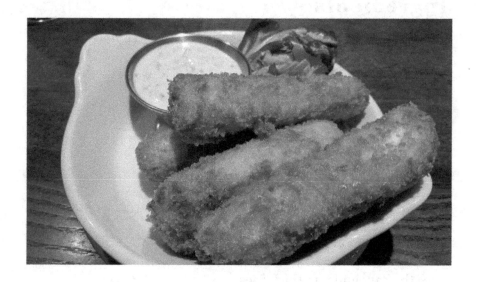

LOW CARB SALMON CAKES

PREP:35 minutes

COOK:15 minutes

TOTAL:50 minutes

Ingredients

1 lb ALDI Fresh Atlantic Salmon Side (half a side)

1/4 Cup Avocado, mashed

1/4 Cup Cilantro, diced + additional for garnish

1 1/2 tsp Yellow curry powder

1/2 tsp l Sea Salt Grinder

1/4 Cup + 4 tsp Tapioca Starch, divided (40g) *Read notes for lower carb version

2 Simply Nature Organic Cage Free Brown Eggs

1/2 Cup Coconut Flakes (30g)

Coconut Oil, melted (for brushing)

For the Greens:

2 tsp Coconut Oil, melted

6 Cups Arugula & Spinach Mix, tightly packed

Pinch of Sea Salt Grinder

Instructions

Remove the skin from the salmon, dice the flesh, and add it into a large bowl.

Add in the avocado, cilantro, curry powder, sea salt and stir until well mixed. Then, stir in 4 tsp of the tapioca starch until well incorporated.

Line a baking sheet with parchment paper. Form the salmon into 8, 1/4 cup-sized patties, just over 1/2 inch thick, and place them onto the pan. Freeze for 20 minutes so they are easier to work with.

While the patties freeze, pre-heat your Air Fryer to 400 degrees for 10 minutes, rubbing the basket with coconut oil. Additionally, whisk the eggs and place them into a shallow plate. Place the remaining 1/4 cup of Tapioca starch and the coconut flakes in separate shallow plates as well.

Once the patties have chilled, dip one into the tapioca starch, making sure it's fully covered. Then, dip it into the egg, covering it entirely, and gently brushing off any excess. Finally, press just the top and sides of the cake into the coconut flakes and place it, coconut flake-side up, into the air fryer. Repeat with all cakes. **

Gently brush the tops with a little bit of melted coconut oil (optional, but recommended) and cook until the outside is golden brown and crispy, and the inside is juicy and tender, about 15 minutes. Note: the patties will stick to the Air Fryer basked a little, so use a sharp-edged spatula to remove them.

When the cakes have about 5 minutes left to cook, heat the coconut oil up in a large pan on medium heat. Add in the Arugula and Spinach Mix, and a pinch of salt, and cook, stirring constantly, until the greens JUST begin to wilt, only 30 seconds - 1 minute.

Divide the greens between 4 plates, followed by the salmon cakes. Garnish with extra cilantro and DEVOUR!

If You Want to Bake In The Oven:

Preheat your oven to 400 degrees and line a baking sheet with parchment paper, placing a cooling rack on top of the pan. Rub the cooling rack with coconut oil.

Place the patties, coconut-side up, onto the cooling rack and bake for 15-17 minutes until crispy. NOTE: we liked these better in the air fryer, as they do get a little crispier, but they are still good in the oven!

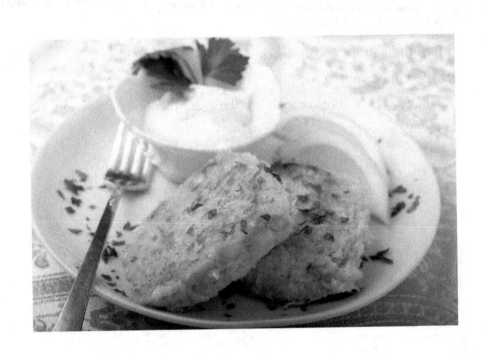

DELICIOUS POTATO CAULIFLOWER PATTIES

Prep Time: 15

Cook Time: 20

Total Time: 35 minutes

Yield: 7

Ingredients

1 medium to large sweet potato, peeled

2 cup cauliflower florets

1 green onion, chopped.

1 tsp minced garlic

2 tbsp organic ranch seasoning mix or dairy seasoning mix of choice

1 cup packed cilantro (fresh)

1/2 tsp chili powder

1/4 tsp cumin

2 tbsp arrowroot starch or gluten free flour of choice

1/4 cup ground flaxseed

1/4 cup sunflower seeds (or pumpkin seeds)

1/4 tsp Kosher Salt and pepper (or to taste)

Dipping sauce of choice

Instructions

Pre-heat oven to 400F. Line a baking sheet (or oil) and set aside.

Next cut your peeled sweet potato into smaller pieces. Place in a food processor or blender and pulse until the larger pieces are broken up.

Add in your cauliflower, onion, and garlic and pulse again.

Add in the sunflower seeds, flaxseed, arrowroot (or flour), cilantro, and remaining seasonings. Pulse or place on medium until a thick batter is formed. See blog for picture.

Place batter in larger bowl. Scoop 1/4 cup of the batter out at a time and form into patties about 1.5 inches thick. Place on baking sheet.

Repeat until you have about 7-10 patties.

Chill in freeze for 10 minutes so the patties can set.

Once set, place patties in oven for 20 minutes, flipping halfway. If you made your patties extra thick, they could take closer to 25 minutes.

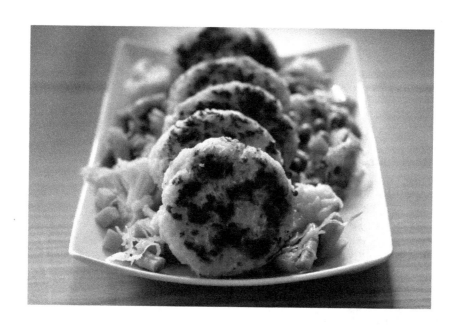

AIR FRYER ITALIAN ZUCCHINI CHIPS

Prep Time15 minutes

Cook Time10 minutes

Total Time25 minutes

Servings5

Ingredients

1 large zucchini Mine weighed 1.5 pounds.

1/2 cup all-purpose flour

1 teaspoon Italian Seasoning

1 teaspoon Smoked Paprika or your favorite seasoning

1/4 cup finely shredded parmesan cheese

salt and pepper to taste

2 eggs, beaten

1 1/2-2 cups breadcrumb I used panko breadcrumbs.

cooking oil spray

Instructions

Spray the air fryer basket with cooking oil.

Add eggs, flour, and breadcrumbs to separate bowls.

Slice the zucchini into chips about 1/4 of an inch thick. You can also use a mandolin for precise slicing. You want to get the zucchini chips all about the same size so that they cook at an even temperature.

Season the flour with salt and pepper to taste, and paprika and add shredded parmesan.

Dip the zucchini in the flour, then egg, and then the breadcrumbs and place in the air fryer. Make sure to coat the chip fully in the eggs so that the breadcrumbs will stick.

Keep a moist towel nearby because your hands will get sticky.

Spray the zucchini chips with cooking oil spray using a spray bottle.

Air Fry for 5 minutes on 400 degrees.

Open and flip the chips. Spray with additional oil and cook for an additional 4-7 minutes on 400 degrees. The zucchini chips will brown by 8 minutes, if you like them crispy, cook them a little longer. Mine were ready around 10-11 minutes.

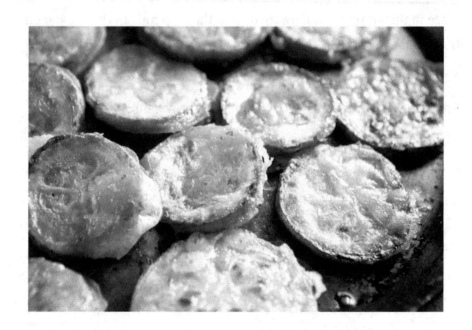

AIR FRYER JUMBO SHRIMP

Ingredients

2 pounds jumbo cooked shrimp, peeled and deveined

4 cloves garlic, minced

2/3 cup parmesan cheese, grated

1 teaspoon pepper

1/2 teaspoon oregano

1 teaspoon basil

1 teaspoon onion powder

2 tablespoons olive oil

Lemon, quartered

Instructions

In a large bowl, combine garlic, parmesan cheese, pepper, oregano, basil, onion powder and olive oil.

Gently toss shrimp in mixture until evenly-coated.

Spray air fryer basket with non-stick spray and place shrimp in basket.

Cook at 350 degrees for 8-10 minutes or until seasoning on shrimp is browned.

Squeeze the lemon over the shrimp before serving.

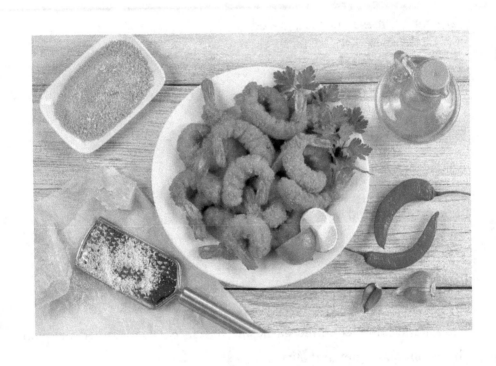

LOW CARB RANCH STEAK NUGGETS

Ingredients

1 pound venison steak or beef steak, cut into chunks.

1 large Egg(s), Organic Pasture Raised

Lard or palm oil for frying

Keto Breading

1/2 cup grated parmesan cheese

1/2 cup pork panko

1/2 teaspoon Homemade Seasoned Salt

Chipotle Ranch Dip

1/4 cup mayonnaise

1/4 cup Sour Cream (organic, cultured)

1+ teaspoon chipotle pastes to taste

1/2 teaspoon Homemade Ranch Dressing & Dip Mix

1/4 medium lime, juiced

Instructions

For the Chipotle Ranch Dip: Combine all ingredients, mix well. 1 teaspoon of chipotle paste yields a medium-spice version, use more or less according to your own taste preferences. I encourage you to use my homemade ranch dressing and dip mix, it's superior to any store brought version. Refrigerate at least 30 minutes before serving, will keep for up to 1 week.

Combine Pork Panko, parmesan cheese and seasoned salt - again use my homemade not the store-bought stuff. Set aside.

Beat 1 egg. place beaten egg 1 bowl and breading mix in another.

Dip chunks of steak in egg, then breading. Place on a wax paper lined sheet pan or plate.

FREEZE breaded raw steak bites for 30 minutes before frying. This helps to ensure that the breading will NOT LIFT when fried.

Heat Lard to roughly 325 degrees F. Working in batches as necessary, fry steak nuggets (from frozen or chilled) until browned, about 2-3 minutes.

Transfer to a paper towel lined plate, season with a sprinkle of salt and serve with Chipotle Ranch.

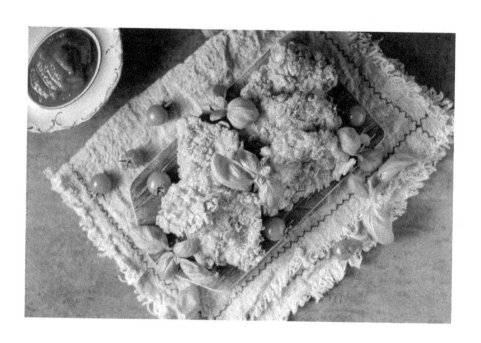

AIR FRYER SALMON FILLETS TERIYAKI

prep time: 5 MINS cook time: 8 MINS marinade: 15 MINS total time: 28 MINS servings: 3

Ingredients

1/3+1/4 cup Keto Teriyaki Sauce, see notes

16.5 oz. salmon fillets (3 slices at 5.5 oz per fillet), 1.5-inch at thickest

1/8 tsp xanthan gum

Toasted white sesame seeds, sprinkle optional

1 bulb scallion, chopped

Instructions

For the teriyaki sauce:

Follow this keto teriyaki sauce recipe instructions to prepare the sauce but do not add the xanthan gum thickener. Let the sauce cool to room temperature.

Teriyaki salmon marinade:

In a small baking tray or casserole dish that's just big enough to fill in all the salmon pieces, pour over ⅓ cup of the teriyaki sauce and marinate the fish skin side up for 15-20 minutes.

Air fried the salmon:

Line the air fryer basket with a thin layer of parchment paper or an air fryer liner. Slightly drip off the marinade and place the fish, side skin down, in the basket and with some gap between the fillets. Discard the marinade.

Air fry at 400F for 7 to 9 minutes. The exact time will depend on the thickness of the fish and your appliance. Mine was done at 7 minutes for medium-rare and 8 minutes for medium.

To thicken the teriyaki sauce, take ¼ cup of the sauce and add it to a small sauce pot. Bring it to a low simmer. Gradually and slowly sprinkle in 1/8 tsp xanthan gum while whisking at the same time to prevent clumps.

Teriyaki homemade sauce in a white and blue cup

The fish will be nearly opaque when cut into, at 120F (49C) at the thickest part. You can peek into the thickest part with a sharp knife or fork. It should flake easily, but still has a little translucency in the center.

Transfer the fishes to a plater. Glaze the salmon with teriyaki sauce. Sprinkle with toasted sesame seeds, if using, and scallions. Remove the skin before serving. I recommend serving them warm.

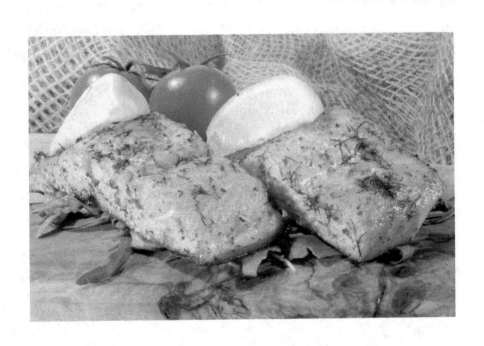

AIR FRYER AVOCADO

Servings: 35 fries

Calories: 46 kcal

Ingredients

2 large avocados

½ cup unsweetened almond milk, may also sub with 1 large egg if not vegan

½ cup superfine blanched almond flour

For the coating:

1 cup unsweetened toasted shredded coconut, OR sub with crushed Simple Mills Grain-Free Sea Salt Almond Flour Crackers (or other favorite grain-free crackers like Hu's Kitchen Grain-Free Crackers)

1.5 tbsp Cajun seasoning spice mix OR smoked paprika

Salt and pepper

For the optional dip:

⅓ cup vegan mayo

1 tbsp lemon juice

½ tbsp Cajun seasoning

Salt and pepper to taste

Instructions

Use a large knife to cut your avocados in half and remove the pit from the middle. Cut the avocado into wedges or "fries".

Homemade Guacamole - this quick and simple recipe is the perfect easy party dip with tortilla chips or along with tacos or by the spoonful. Best of all, only 6 ingredients to make for your next Mexican-inspired meal.

Oven Method

Preheat oven to 400F. Line a large baking sheet with parchment paper.

Gather three wide shallow bowls. Place the almond milk in one bowl, the almond flour in the next bowl and combine the coating ingredients in the the third bowl.

Take one avocado slice, place it in the flour. Make sure it is fully coated in flour then gently shake to get rid of any excess flour.

Place it in the almond milk and again make sure it is fully coated and wet. You will find it easier if you use one hand for the first two steps and then the other hand for the breading, so you don't get too messy!

Finally place it in the coconut breading, making sure it is fully coated, then place on the baking pan.

Repeat until all the slices are coated. Place the baking sheet in the oven for 15-20 minutes until turning golden brown.

FOR THE DIP:

Make the dip by mixing all the ingredients together. Enjoy with the avocado fries!

Air Fryer Method

Place the breaded avocado sticks in a single layer in the air fryer basket, you will have to work in batches.

Lightly coat with cooking spray and cook for 8-12 minutes at 375F, or until golden and crispy, flipping halfway through.

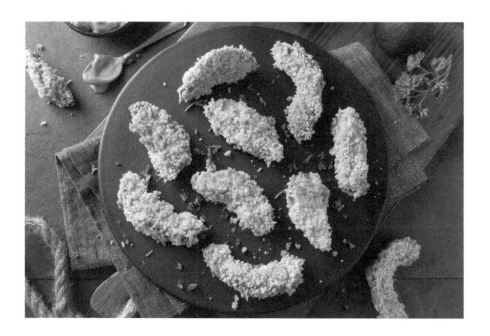

Creamy Chicken, Rice, And Peas

Preparation Time: 10 minutes Cooking Time: 30 minutes Servings: 4

Ingredients

1 lb. chicken breasts

1 cup white rice

Salt and black pepper

1 tbsp. olive oil

Three garlic cloves

One yellow onion

½ cup white wine

¼ cup heavy cream

1 cup chicken stock

¼ cup parsley

2 cups peas

One and ½ cups parmesan

Directions:

Spice chicken breasts with pepper and salt, sprinkle half oil over them. Rub well and place in the air fryer, then cook at 360 °F for 6 minutes.

Heat pan with remaining oil over high heat. Add garlic, wine, onion, stock, pepper, and heavy cream, salt, stir, simmer, and cook for 9 minutes.

Put chicken breasts in a heatproof dish and add peas, cream mix, rice, and toss. Sprinkle parsley and parmesan all over, put in the air fryer, and cook at 420 °F for 10 minutes.

Divide between plates and serve hot while.

AIR FRYER KETO QUESO FUNDIDO

Prep Time: 10 minutes Cook Time: 25 minutes Stand Time: 30 minutes
Total Time: 35 minutes

Ingredients

4 ounces (113.4 g) Mexican-style chorizo, casings removed

1 cup (160 g) onions, chopped

1 tablespoon (1 tablespoon) Minced Garlic

1 cup (149 g) diced tomatoes

2 (2) jalepenos, diced

2 teaspoons (2 teaspoons) Ground Cumin

2 cups (473.18 g) grated Oaxaca cheese or Mozzarella

1/2 cup (121 g) Half and Half

Instructions

In a 6 x 3 heatproof pan, mix together the chorizo, onion, garlic, tomatoes, jalepenos and ground cumin. Place pan in the air fryer basket.

Set the air fryer to 400F for 15 minutes or until the sausage is cooked. Halfway through cooking, stir the mixture to break up the sausage.

Add the cheese and half and half and stir again.

Set air fryer to 320F for 10 minutes until the cheese has melted.

Serve with tortillas or chips.

To further reduce carbs, cut onions in half, and use cherry tomatoes instead of regular tomatoes

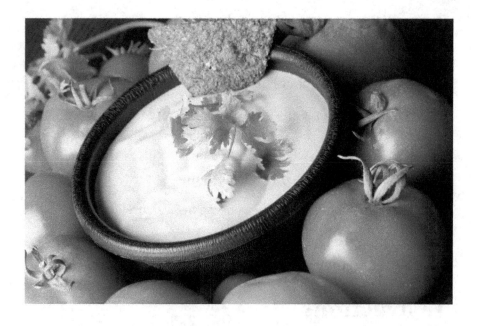

AIR FRYER TILAPIA FILLETS

Prep Time: 10

Cook Time: 8

Total Time: 18

Yield: 4 servings

Ingredients

1 teaspoon lemon juice

1 teaspoon dried oregano

1 teaspoon garlic powder

1 teaspoon salt

4 (6 ounces) tilapia fillets

olive oil spray

Instructions

Start by making the rub, mix together the lemon juice, oregano, garlic powder, and salt.

Then rub the spices onto the fish. (Both sides)

Spray the fish with olive oil spray, and then place into the air fryer basket or oven. Set the temperature for 400 degrees F, for 4 minutes, after 4 minutes, flip (spray again) and add another 4 minutes.

Plate, serve, and enjoy!

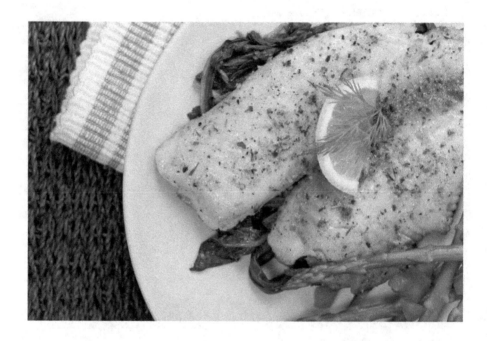

AIR FRYER FLANK STEAK WITH CHIMICHURRI SAUCE

Prep Time: 10

Cook Time: 10

Total Time: 20

Yield: 4 servings

Ingredients

2 pounds flank steak

Chimichurri Sauce:

1/2 cup diced parsley

1/2 cup diced cilantro

1/2 onion

1 teaspoon salt

1/2 teaspoon black pepper

1 teaspoon garlic

1/2 teaspoon red pepper flakes

1/3 cup olive oil

2 tablespoons red wine vinegar

Instructions

The first thing I do when making steak, let the meat rest at room temperature for AT LEAST 30 minutes.

Start by preheating the air fryer, steak is one of the few recipes, that I preheat the air fryer for. But the meat will come out better, so turn the air fryer oven'/basket on for 5 minutes at 400 degrees F.

Then rub the olive oil or butter all over the steak, and season with salt and pepper.

Set the steaks in the air fryer for 6 minutes, then flip and air fry for another 6 minutes.

Again, per Bobby Flay, let the steak rest for at least 5 minutes.

Plate, serve, and enjoy!

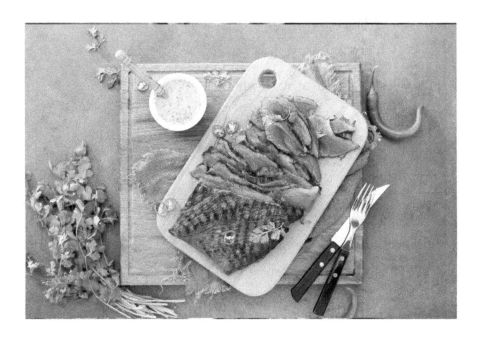

AIR FRYER SCALLOPS WITH TOMATO CREAM SAUCE

Prep Time: 5 minutes Cook Time: 10 minutes Total Time: 15 minutes

Servings: 2

Ingredients

3/4 cup (178.5 g) Heavy Whipping Cream

1 tablespoon (1 tablespoon) Tomato Paste

1 tablespoon (1 tablespoon) chopped fresh basil

1 teaspoon (1 teaspoon) Minced Garlic

1/2 teaspoon (0.5 teaspoon) Kosher Salt

1/2 teaspoon (0.5 teaspoon) Ground Black Pepper

1 12 oz (1 12 oz) Frozen Spinach, thawed and drained

8 (8) jumbo sea scallops

Cooking Oil Spray

additional salt and pepper to season scallops

Instructions

Spray a 7-inch heatproof pan, and place the spinach in an even layer at the bottom.

Spray both sides of the scallops with vegetable oil, sprinkle a little more salt and pepper on them, and place scallops in the pan on top of the spinach.

In a small bowl, mix together the cream, tomato paste, basil, garlic, salt and pepper and pour over the spinach and scallops.

Set the air fryer to 350F for 10 minutes until the scallops are cooked through to an internal temperature of 135F and the sauce is hot and bubbling. Serve immediately.

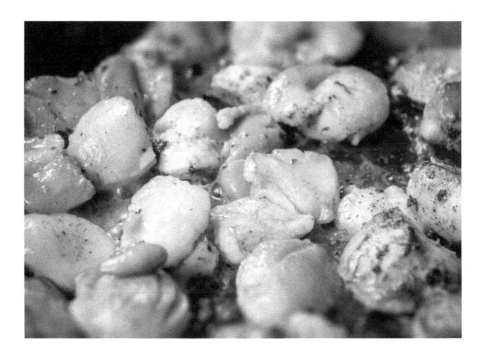

CRISPY AIR FRYER BRUSSELS SPROUTS

Prep Time

5 mins

Cook Time

15 mins

Total Time

20 mins

Servings: 4 servings Calories: 155kcal

Ingredients

2 cups Brussel sprouts

2 Tablespoons coconut oil

1/4 cup parmesan cheese grated

1/4 cup almonds sliced and crushed

2 Tablespoons everything bagel seasoning

Sea salt to taste

Instructions

Add Brussel sprouts to a medium saucepan with 2 cups of water, cover and cook over medium heat for 8-10 minutes.

Drain Brussels sprouts and allow to cool, then slice each one in half.

Toss Brussel sprouts in a large mixing bowl with oil, parmesan cheese, crushed almonds, everything bagel seasoning, and salt.

If needed, use a wooden spoon to stir and make sure the Brussel sprouts are fully coated in seasoning.

Transfer the Brussels sprouts to the air fryer, and cook for 12 to 15 minutes at 375 or until golden for both sides.

Notes

Note: Nutrition information is a rough estimate only; actual values will vary based on the exact ingredients used and amount of recipe prepared.

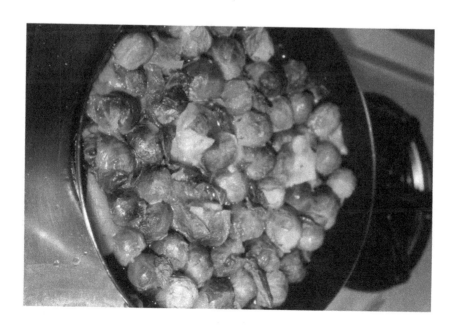

AIR FRYER VEGETABLE CHIPS

Preparation time 10 min.

Baking time 15 min.

Total time 25 min.

Ingredients

200 g parsnips

and or

200 g carrots

and or

2 pieces of beetroot

Spices as desired (e.g. sals, paprika powder, chilli, rosemary, etc.)

Preparation

Preheat the air fryer to 180 degrees for about 3 minutes.

Cut the vegetables, preferably with a vegetable slicer, into thin slices.

Since the different types of vegetables take different times in the air fryer to become crispy, you should prepare each one individually.

Parsnip chips: Place the thin parsnip slices in the basket of the hot air fryer and deep-fry them at 180 degrees for about 15 minutes.

Carrot chips: Place the thin carrot slices in the basket of the hot air fryer and deep-fry them at 180 degrees for about 20 minutes.

Beetroot chips: Place the thin beetroot slices in the basket of the hot air fryer and deep-fry them at 180 degrees for about 25 minutes.

To ensure that the vegetable chips are crispy on all sides, you should take the frying basket out of the hot air fryer about every 5 minutes and shake it well.

It is best to enjoy the vegetable chips straight away, as they will no longer be as crispy after a while.

After the vegetable chips are crispy, they can be refined with salt, paprika powder, chilli, rosemary or other spices, for example

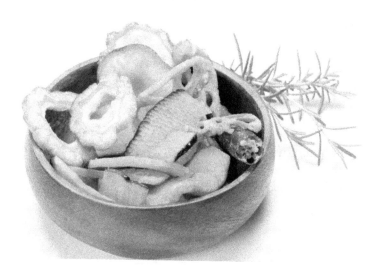

AIR FRYER CINNAMON QUARK BALLS

Preparation time: 5 Mins Cooking time: 30 Mins Total time: 35 Mins

ingredients

300 grams of curd

300 grams of flour 405

3 teaspoons of tartar baking powder

3 eggs

70 grams of sugar

½ teaspoon cinnamon

1 pinch of salt

a large pinch of ground vanilla

Mixture of sugar and cinnamon

Liquid butter

Preparation

Put the quark, salt, sugar, eggs, cinnamon, vanilla in the mixing bowl and mix for 35 seconds / speed 4.

Add baking powder and flour and add 2 minutes / kneading setting.

Either fry the quark balls in hot fat or use the Air fryer.

Preheat this to 180 degrees.

Use an ice cream scoop to put a large blob on the grill plate (please oil a little beforehand).

Bake the quark balls for 8 minutes at 180 degrees, then turn them over and another 3 minutes

With the amount of dough, you have to bake 3 times.

Then pour liquid butter on the quark balls and roll in the sugar-cinnamon mixture

Best to enjoy lukewarm.

Update: It is also possible in the oven: 180 degrees for 15 minutes!

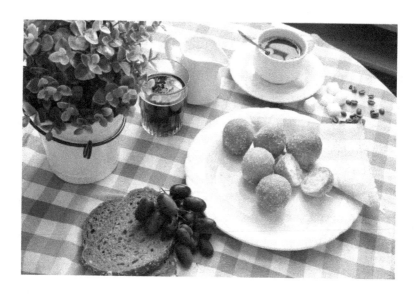

OVEN GREEN CURRY DRUMSTICKS

ingredient list

2 tablespoons (32 g)

green curry paste

1 tsp freshly grated ginger

2 tablespoons (8 g) fresh coriander

1/4 tsp Himalayan

salt

1/8 tsp Cayenne pepper

1/4 cup unsweetened full-fat yogurt or unsweetened non-dairy yogurt

2 tablespoons (30 ml) avocado oil

6th Chicken legs

Instructions

Mix the green curry paste, ginger, coriander, salt, cayenne pepper, yoghurt and oil in a food processor and stir until smooth. Pour the marinade into a large glass bowl and add the drumsticks; throw to coat well. Cover the bowl and put it in the refrigerator for 3 hours or overnight.

Preheat the oven to 230 °C, line a large baking sheet with foil and place a well-oiled grid in the pan. Place the marinated drumsticks on the prepared rack and put the pan in the oven for 45 minutes. Turn the drumsticks over halfway. At the end of the cooking time, turn the oven on roast and cook for another 3 to 5 minutes or until the drumsticks appear crispy. Take the pan out of the oven and let the drumsticks cool down a bit before serving. The drumsticks can be stored covered in the refrigerator for up to 3 days.

Substitutions: To make this recipe dairy-free or paleo, use unsweetened dairy-free yogurt. To make this recipe vegetarian, use paneer or tofu in place of chicken

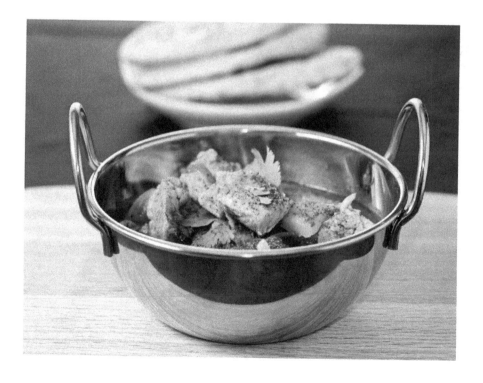

AIR FRYER VEGAN CHICKEN WINGS

preparation   10 Minutes

cooking time 50 Minutes

waiting period 50 Minutes

Servings   2 people

ingredient list

1 large cauliflower

100 G Chickpea flour or wheat flour

180 ml unsweetened soy or almond milk

60 ml water

2 Tl Garlic powder

1 1/2 Tl noble sweet paprika powder

salt

pepper

70 G Panko flour

250 ml Grill & Tex Mex Sauce

2 two spring onions

vegan aioli from Byodo for dipping

Sriracha sauce (optional)

Vegan chicken wings made from cauliflower

Instructions

Preheat the oven to 180 ° C.

In a large bowl, mix the flour, vegetable milk, water, garlic powder, paprika powder, salt and pepper.

Divide / cut the cauliflower into bite-sized florets. Dip the cauliflower florets in the flour mixture so that they are completely covered. The cauliflower wings also taste great when you add them to panko flour before baking. Panko flour is a breadcrumb from Japanese cuisine that gets really nice and crispy. Line a baking sheet with parchment paper and distribute the cauliflower florets evenly on it. Do not lay on top of each other. Bake for 25 minutes.

Take the cauliflower out of the oven after 25 minutes and dip it in the Tex-Mex sauce or, alternatively, spread it evenly over the cauliflower florets. If you want the vegan cauliflower wings a little hotter, you can spread a little Sriracha sauce over them. Bake again for 25 minutes.

Cut the spring onions into rings and spread over the vegan cauliflower chicken wings. Serve with the vegan aioli.

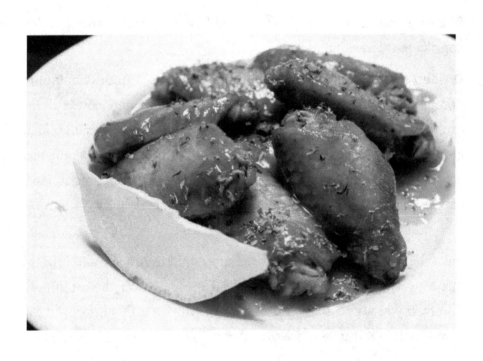

AIR FRYER BROCCOLI

Preparation time: 10 min

Preparation time: 30 min

Total time: 40 min

Servings: 10

Ingredients

1 broccoli

4 eggs

100 gr almond flour

1/2 tsp sea salt

2 pinches of black pepper

optional: dried herbs for it

Instructions

Preheat the oven to 175°C

Chop the broccoli into rice with the pulse function of your food processor. You can also use a food chopper or chop the broccoli by hand.

Beat the eggs in a mixing bowl. Add the broccoli rice, almond flour, sea salt and black pepper. Mix into a thick dough

Spoon the dough onto a baking tray covered with parchment paper. Use a spatula to spread the dough until it is about 1/2 inch thick.

Bake for 30 minutes or more until golden brown

Let it cool for at least 10 minutes. Turnover and remove the parchment paper. Cut it into square pieces and keep it in a large glass jar in the refrigerator

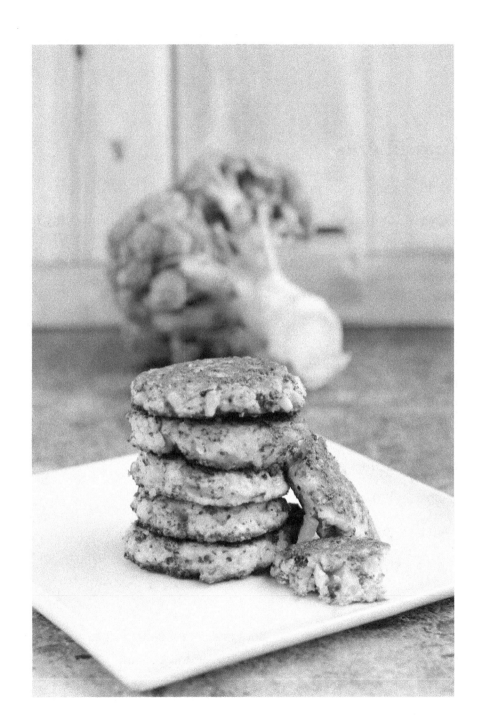

AIR FRYER BLISSFUL SALMON

Ingredients

For the fish (per person):

1 slice of (defrosted) salmon - wild salmon because of the healthy fats, MSC quality mark because of the responsible fishing

pepper and salt or fish seasoning, to taste

2-3 slices of bacon

1 tbsp pesto

1-2 sprigs of thyme (preferably lemon thyme)

20 g feta

For with it (per person):

2 snack tomatoes

pepper, salt, 1 basil leaf

1 tsp pine nuts

To step

Per person:

Sprinkle the salmon steak on both sides with salt and pepper or with fish herbs. Massage the herbs in a little with your hand.

Place the bacon slices on a plate. For the largest salmon steak, I used 3 slices, for the rest 2 was sufficient.

Spread half of the pesto on the bottom of the salmon steak and then place it with the pesto side on the bacon. The salmon has been turned over for the photo.

Then spread the rest of the pesto on top. Crumble the feta over it. Remove the leaves from the thyme and sprinkle them over the feta.

Wrap the bacon around the salmon.

Finishing and baking:

Preheat the Air fryer to 180 degrees Celsius.

Halve the snack tomatoes. This is easiest with a serrated / tomato knife. It is easy if they stay together on the side, then they do not wobble. Cut the basil leaves into strips. Sprinkle salt and pepper and the basil strips over the tomatoes and place them between the salmon steaks.

Sprinkle the pine nuts over the dish.

Place the dish in the Airfyrer for about 15 minutes, or until the bacon is nice and crispy. And then... feast!

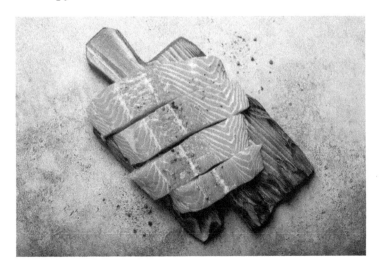

AIR FRYER BROCCOLI

Prep Time: 2 minutes

Cook Time: 8 minutes

0 minutes

Total Time: 10 minutes

Servings: 2 servings

Ingredients

3-4 cups broccoli florets

2 tablespoons olive oil

1/4 teaspoon garlic powder

1/4 teaspoon salt

1/4 teaspoon pepper

Instructions

Add broccoli, olive oil, garlic powder, salt & pepper to a large bowl and toss to combine.

Transfer to air fryer and set to 375F for 8 minutes. Shake halfway through.

Once the timer goes off, remove and serve immediately.

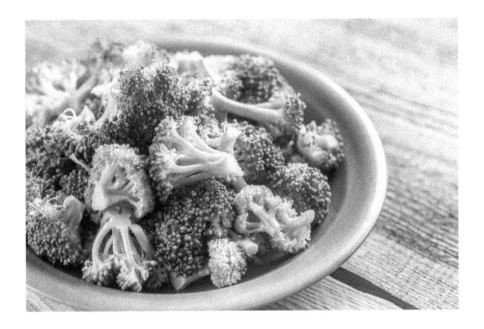

AIR FRYER CAULIFLOWER CROQUETTES!

Ingredients

6 croquettes

1.2 khd per croquette

300 g of cauliflower

75 g parmesan cheese

1 egg

1/2 tsp paprika

2 sprigs of chopped coriander

pepper

50 g bacon

15 g parmesan cheese

Preparation method:

Cut the cauliflower into florets and cook them al dente. Puree the cauliflower and squeeze the excess moisture from the cauliflower puree with a kitchen towel.

Mix the cauliflower puree with the parmesan cheese, egg, paprika, coriander and pepper and make 6 croquettes.

Chop the bacon with a food processor and add the parmesan cheese.

(if you don't like bacon, you can also use only parmesan cheese or finely ground low-carb crackers)

Put the croquettes through the finely ground bacon and parmesan cheese and put them in the airfryer at 180c for 10 minutes.

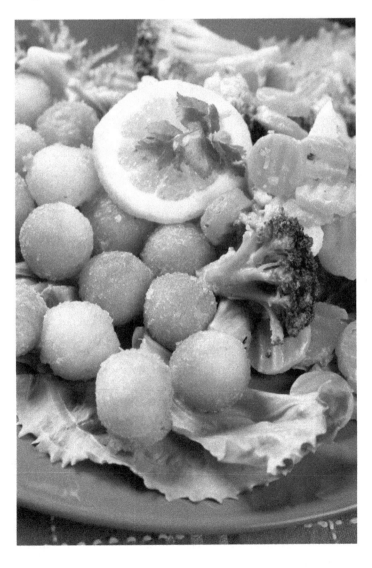

AIR FRYER CRISPY TOFU

Prep: 30 minutes Cook: 15 minutes Total: 45 minutes servings: 4

Ingredients

1 16-oz block extra-firm tofu 453 g

2 Tbsp soy sauce 30 mL

1 Tbsp toasted sesame oil* 15 mL

1 Tbsp olive oil 15 mL

1 clove garlic minced

Instructions

Press: Press tofu for at least 15 minutes, using either a or by setting a heavy pan on top of it, letting the moisture drain. When finished, cut tofu into bite-sized blocks and transfer to a bowl.

Flavor: Combine all remaining ingredients in a small bowl. Drizzle over tofu and toss to coat. Let tofu marinate for an additional 15 minutes.

Air Fry: Preheat your air fryer to 375 degrees F (190 C). Add tofu blocks to your air fryer basket in a single layer. Cook for 10 to 15 minutes, shaking the pan occasionally to promote even cooking.

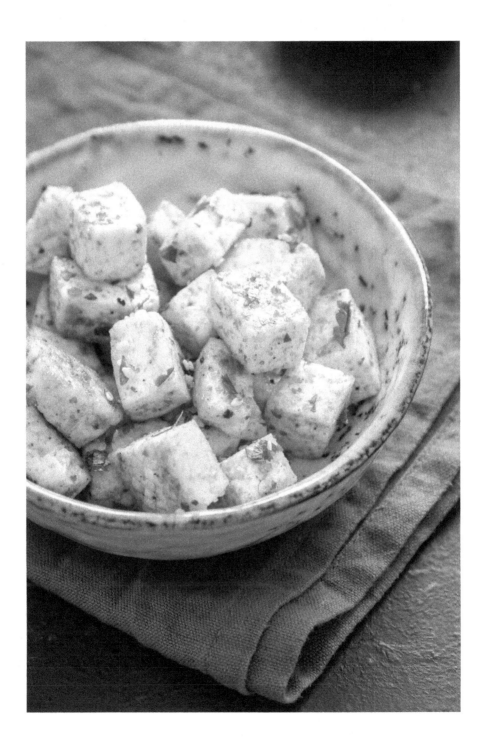

AIR FRYER BEEF KOFTA KABAB

Prep Time: 10 minutes Cook Time: 10 minutes Total Time: 20 minutes servings: 4

Ingredients

1 tablespoon (1 tablespoon) Oil

1 pound (453.59 g) Lean Ground Beef

¼ cup (15 g) Chopped Parsley

1 tablespoon (1 tablespoon) Minced Garlic

2 tablespoons (2 tablespoons) kofta kabab spice mix

1 teaspoon (1 teaspoon) Kosher Salt

Instructions

Using a stand mixer, blend together all ingredients. If you have time, let the mixture sit in the fridge for 30 minutes. You can also mix it up and set aside for a day or two until you're ready to make the kababs

Although I tried this with and without skewers, it really makes no difference to the final product. Since it's a lot easier to simply shape the kababs by hand, divide the meat into four and make four long sausage shapes (or Pokémon shape or whatever you want).

Place the kababs in your air fryer and cook at 370F for 10 minutes.

Check with a meat thermometer to ensure that the kababs have an internal temperature of 145F.

Sprinkle with additional parsley for garnishing and serve with tzatziki, a cucumber tomato salad, and pita bread.

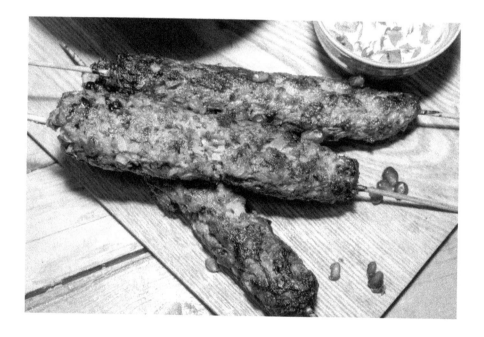

AIRFRYER HEALTHY SANDWICH

Ingredients

4 slices of white floor bread

4 slices of Gouda young matured

2 slices of roasted ham

15 g unsalted butter in the tub

Instructions

Preheat the airfryer to 180 ° C. Cover a slice of bread successively with a slice of cheese, slice of ham and another slice of cheese. Cover with a slice of bread. Make another sandwich like this.

Spread the outside of the sandwich with half the butter. Bake 1 sandwich in the airfryer for 5 minutes until golden brown. Turn halfway through. Bake another sandwich in this way.

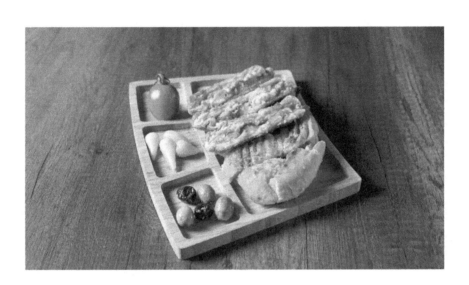

VEGETABLE PAPRIKA CHIPS

Servings 5,

Cooking time: 15-20 minutes

Ingredients

1 small parsnip

3 carrots (suggestion: take three different colored carrots)

¼ celeriac

¼ swede

1 tablespoon of paprika

½ teaspoon of garlic powder

½ teaspoon chili powder

Pinch of salt

3 eggs

1 tablespoon of mustard

100 grams of Panko

250ml Greek yogurt 0%

2 cloves of garlic

3 tablespoons of freshly chopped chives

Instructions

Bring a pan with water and some salt to the boil. Wash all vegetables and then peel them. Cut thick fries and blanch them briefly. Rinse with cold water and drain well.

Beat the eggs with the spices and mix it all the way through the sliced vegetable fries. Now sprinkle the panko over the wet fries and mix well with your hands.

Cover the bottom of the basket with the chips, but make sure it is not overfilled. Bake the fries for 15 to 20 minutes at 180 degrees. Shake them twice in between.

Make the yogurt sauce while baking. Cut the chives and squeeze the garlic cloves and mix them with the yogurt. Season with salt and pepper from the mill. Then serve the fries with the yoghurt sauce

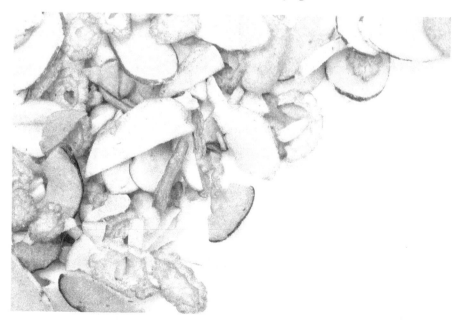

ZUCCHINI AND CHEESE BREAD

Ingredients

1 tbsp olive oil

1 onion

2 cloves of garlic

100 gr ham

450 g zucchini

200 gr feta

200 gr ricotta

40 gr grated old cheese

6 sprigs of thyme

60 gr green olives without stone

6 eggs

150 g spelled bread flour (or regular flour, that is also possible)

Instructions

Preheat the oven to 180 degrees (electric) or 160 degrees (hot air). Grease a 20x30cm baking pan with butter. And then cover with baking paper.

Finely chop the onion and garlic, put the olive oil in a frying pan and fry the onion and garlic on low heat for 3-5 minutes until golden brown.

Grate the zucchini. Chop the olives roughly and crumble the feta. Put everything in a large bowl and add the ricotta and grated old cheese. Spoon the onion and garlic into the mixture. Remove the leaves from the thyme sprigs and add. Cut the ham into strips and add some salt to the mixture.

Stir the eggs, add the flour and stir until it becomes a smooth mixture. Add to the zucchini mix and stir well.

Spoon the mixture into the baking tin and smooth the top. Bake for 40-50 minutes or until the top is golden brown. Prick the courgetti bread with a wooden skewer to see if the bread is cooked properly. The skewer must come out of the bread dry. If not, put it back in the oven. Cut the bread into 10 pieces.

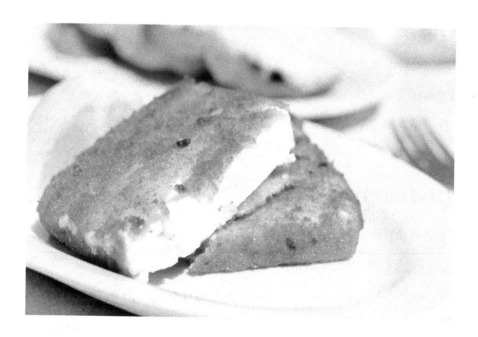

LOW CARB PARMESAN BREAD

Ingredients

Based on 2 people

Parmesan grated

5 tbsp

almond flour

3 tbsp

baking powder

½ tsp

melted butter

1 tbsp

1 egg

Instructions

Mix all dry ingredients in a bowl.

Add egg and butter and mix all ingredients.

Divide the dough between a few buttered coffee cups or in a muffin tin.

You can quickly prepare this in the microwave. Then they are ready in 3 to 5 minutes

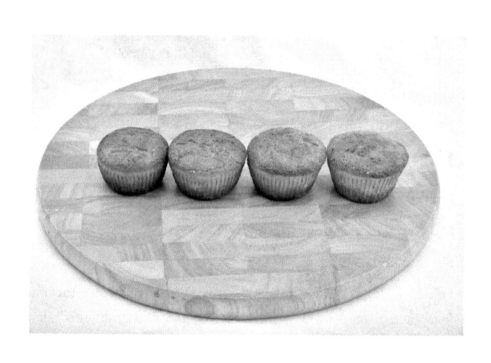

AIRFRYER CINNAMON CARROT CAKE

Ingredients

140 g Soft brown sugar

2 eggs, beaten

140 g butter

1 orange, zest & juice

200 g self-raising flour

1 tsp ground cinnamon

175 g grated carrot, (approx. 2 medium carrots)

60 g sultana

Instructions

Preheat air fryer to 160C.

In a bowl, cream together the butter and sugar.

Slowly add the beaten eggs.

Fold in the flour, a little bit at a time, mixing it as you go. Add the orange juice and zest, grated carrots and sultanas. Gently mix all the ingredients together.

Grease the baking tin and pour the mixture in.

Place baking tin in the air fryer basket and cook for 30 minutes. Check and see if the cake has cooked - use a cocktail stick or metal skewer to poke in the middle. If it comes out wet then cook it for a little longer.

Remove the baking tin from the airfryer basket and allow to cool for 10 minutes before removing from the basket.

AIR FRYER ALMOND CHICKEN

Prep time: 10 mins

Ingredients

Marinade

2 lbs. chicken breast tenders, cut into small pieces

2 cups almond milk

1 tsp salt

½ tsp black pepper

½ ground paprika

Dry Ingredients

3 cups flour

3 tsp salt

2 tsp black pepper

2 tsp paprika

oil spray

Instructions

In a large Ziplock bag, add the chicken and all of the marinade ingredients. Marinate in the refrigerator for at least 2 hours, up to 6 hours.

In a large shallow bowl, add all of the dry ingredients.

After marinating, place chicken and marinade into a large bowl. Working in small batches, dredge chicken chunks into dry ingredients, shake off excess flour, dunk again briefly into the marinade, then dredge for a second time in the dry ingredients, fully coating each piece of chicken. Be sure to gently shake off excess flour mixture.

Spray olive oil onto the bottom and sides of the inside of the air fryer vessel. Place breaded chicken in an even layer; set aside the rest of the chicken. Give the tops of the chicken in the air fryer vessel a quick spray with olive oil, then place into the air fryer.

Air fry at 370°F for 10 minutes. Halfway through this cooking time (at 5 minutes), open the air fryer and shake the basket. If using a tray-style air fryer, use tongs to turn chicken pieces over. Spray tops of chicken with cooking spray, then resume air frying for the remaining 5 minutes.

NOTE: depending on the size and amount of chicken, you may need to allow yours to cook in the air fryer for 2-3 minutes more.

Remove from the air fryer, and repeat steps until you're finished with all of the chicken (usually 3 to 4 batches for me; it may be more or less for you, depending on your air fryer and also how you cut your chicken pieces).

Serve immediately with your favorite dipping sauces. Place any extra chicken into freezer-safe plastic bags and freeze for up to 3 months.

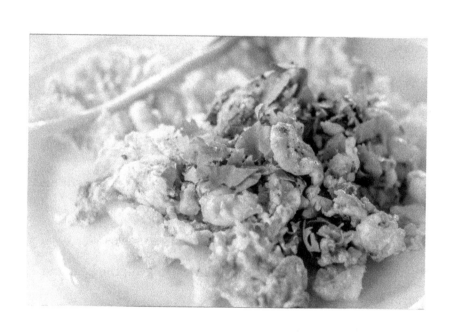

DUCK BREAST SAUCE

Preparation Time: 10 minutes Cooking Time: 32 minutes

Servings: 2

Ingredients

Two duck breasts

1 tbsp. butter

1-star anise

1 tbsp. olive oil

One shallot

9 oz. red plumps

2 tbsp. sugar

2 tbsp. red wine

1 cup beef stock

Directions:

Heat a pan over medium heat with the olive oil, add shallot, stir and cook for 5 minutes,

Add sugar and plums, stir and cook until sugar dissolves.

Add stock and wine, stir, cook for 15 minutes, take off the heat and keep warm for now.

Score duck breasts, season with salt and pepper, rub with melted butter, transfer to a heatproof dish that fits your air fryer, add star anise and plum sauce, introduce in your air fryer and cook at 360 degrees F for 12 minutes.

Divide everything among plates and serve.

TASTY CRISPY CHICKEN BREASTS

Preparation Time: 15 minutes Cooking Time: 12 minutes Servings: 6

Ingredients:

1 cup panko breadcrumbs

½ cup Parmesan cheese, grated

¼ cup fresh rosemary, minced

¼ tsp. cayenne pepper

Salt and ground black pepper, as required

6 (4-ounce) boneless, skinless chicken breasts

3 tbsps. olive oil

Olive oil cooking spray

Directions:

In a shallow dish, add the breadcrumbs, Parmesan cheese, rosemary, cayenne pepper, salt, and black pepper and mix well.

Rub the chicken breasts with oil and then coat with the breadcrumbs mixture evenly.

Arrange the chicken breasts onto the steak tray and spray with cooking spray.

Select "Air Fry" of Air Fryer Oven and then adjust the temperature to 350 degrees F.

Set the timer for 12 minutes and press "Start/Stop" to begin cooking.

When the unit beeps to show that it is preheated, insert the steak tray in the Air fryer Oven.

Flip the chicken breasts once halfway through.

If the cooking time is complete, remove the chicken breasts from Air fryer Oven and serve hot.

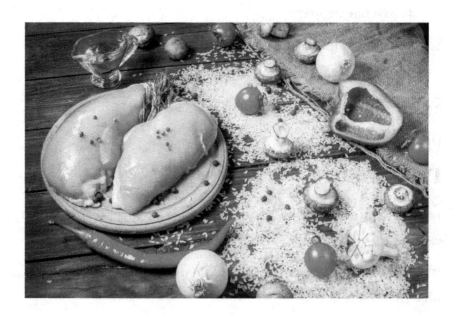

PAPRIKA CHICKEN TENDERS

Preparation Time: 5 minutes Cooking Time: 12 minutes Servings: 4

Ingredients:

1 pound (454 g) chicken tenders

1 tsp. kosher salt

1 tsp. black pepper

½ tsp. smoked paprika

¼ cup coarse mustard

2tbsps. honey

1 cup finely crushed pecans

Directions:

Press Start/Cancel. Preheat the air fryer oven, set the temperature to 350°F (177°C).

Place the chicken in a large bowl. Sprinkle with salt, pepper, and paprika. Toss until the spices are mixed with the chicken. Add the mustard and honey and toss until the chicken is coated.

Place the pecans on a plate. Roll the chicken into the pecans until both sides are coated, dealing with one piece of chicken at a time. Lightly brush off any loose pecans. Place the chicken in the fry basket. Insert at a low position.

Select Bake, Convection, and set time to 12 minutes or until the chicken be cooked through and the pecans are golden brown.

Serve warm.

CHICKEN THIGHS WITH PEANUTS

Preparation Time: 10 minutes Cooking Time: 20 minutes Servings: 6

Ingredients:

½ cup unsweetened full-fat coconut milk

2 tbsps. yellow curry paste

1 tbsp. minced fresh ginger

1 tbsp. minced garlic

1 tsp. kosher salt

1 pound or (454 g) boneless, skinless chicken thighs, halved crosswise

2 tbsps. chopped peanuts

Directions:

In a large bowl, stir together the coconut milk, curry paste, ginger, garlic, and salt until well blended. Add the chicken; toss well to coat. Marinate for 30 minutes and cover or refrigerate for up to 24 hours.

Press Start/Cancel. Preheat the air fryer oven to 375°F (191°C).

Place the chicken (along with marinade) in a baking pan. Place the pan in the fry basket. Insert at a low position.

Select Bake, Convection, and set time to 20 minutes, turning the chicken halfway through the cooking time. Use a meat thermometer to ensure the chicken has reached an internal temperature of 165°F (74°C).

Sprinkle with the chopped peanuts over the chicken and serve.

SIMPLE CHICKEN THIGHS

Preparation Time: 10 minutes Cooking Time: 35 minutes Servings: 6

Ingredients

Six chicken thighs

2 tsp. poultry seasoning

2 tbsp. olive oil

Pepper

Salt

Directions

Insert wire rack in rack position 6. Select bake, set temperature 390 f, timer for 40 minutes. Press start to preheat the oven.

Brush chicken with oil and rub with poultry seasoning, pepper, and salt.

Arrange chicken on roasting pan and bake for 35-40 minutes or until internal temperature reaches 165 f.

Serve and enjoy. Nutrition: Calories319 kcal

BBQ CHICKEN WINGS

Preparation Time: 10 minutes Cooking Time: 55 minutes Servings: 8

Ingredients

32 chicken wings

1 1/2 cups BBQ sauce

1/4 cup olive oil

Pepper

Salt

Directions

Line baking sheet using parchment paper and set aside.

Insert wire rack in rack position 6. Select bake, set temperature 375 f, timer for 55 minutes. Press start to preheat the oven.

In a mixing bowl, toss chicken wings with olive oil, pepper, and salt.

Arrange chicken wings on a baking sheet and bake for 50 minutes.

Toss chicken wings with BBQ sauce and bake for 5 minutes more.

Serve and enjoy

ORANGE JUICE MARINATED STEAK

Preparation Time: 6 minutes Cooking Time: 60 minutes Servings: 4

Ingredients

¼ cup orange juice

1 tsp. ground cumin

2 pounds skirt steak, trimmed from excess fat

2 tbsps. lime juice

2 tbsps. olive oil

Four cloves of garlic, minced

Salt and pepper to taste

Directions:

Put all ingredients in a mixing bowl and allow to marinate in the fridge for at least 2 hours

Preheat the air fryer oven to 390°F.

Place the grill pan accessory in the air fryer.

Grill for 15 minutes per batch and flip the beef every 8 minutes for even grilling.

Meanwhile, pour the marinade on a saucepan and allow to simmer for 10 minutes or until the sauce thickens.

Slice the beef and pour over the sauce.

Conclusion

We have come to the conclusion of this journey into the taste of fried food but in a healthy way. If you picked up this book I imagine you already have an air fryer, but if not, I'm sure you'll soon have this marvel in your kitchen. Having an air fryer in your home is an added value that is becoming more and more popular.

Now you have the ideas for cooking, all that's left to do is start putting them into practice.

Enjoy!!!

Thank you for reading this cookbook

Violet H. Scott